Running Barefoot: The Complete Course

Copyright & Disclaimer

Dedication

To Ken Saxton and the community he has built
Runningbarefoot.org

A Note on Design

This is a dense book. There is a lot of text on every page, with no giant page sized pictures or designs squeezed into the margins. And while I'd like to have that, I don't think it serves you or adds to your learning experience. This book is designed to deliver information, not wow you with visuals. Take notes, write in the margins, and let this book grow with you.

Table of Contents

Now, it is time to Begin, at the Beginning

Starting slow (which may mean walking, or standing barefoot for some of you tenderfoots), and easy, and focusing on learning to run safely, and efficiently, as described in this section, also gives your feet time to become conditioned. It is, as has been said by so many others, absolutely silly to run long distances until after our running technique has been sorted out. After all, you wouldn't want to race your car, if the mechanic had not finished aligning your tires! Why would you do worse to your own body?

If one considers for a moment, that we really, not a single person in the entire world, are designed to run with shoes blocking the sensation of our feet touching the ground while we run, then we might begin to realize, that if the way we are running is uncomfortable while barefoot, that it is not because we are barefoot, but, because we are not running the way we are designed to run.

The main reason we "need" shoes for running, in fact, is not because of modern surfaces, which are not as hard as many natural solid granite trails

We really only need shoes like any drug addict "needs" his/her fix, we have LEARNED to "need" shoes. Our feet have become weak and lazy, due to constant support and "protection".

So you can expect a period of extreme difficulty and discomfort when kicking the shoe habit. Your feet will be growing stronger, from the exercise they have been deprived of for all those years or decades in foot coffins. Your soles have become ultra-sensitive in a desperate attempt to feel the sensation of touching the ground through the thick soles of your shoes, whose main or "sole" purpose was to prevent your soles from feeling the ground!

So, expect some pain, some intense stimulation, and a great deal of adjustment. But, don't fear, for most fears are way over-exaggerated. Yes, you will step on things. Yes there will be some occasional cuts, bruises, etc.. In most cases, these injuries are not the end of the world. In fact, in most cases, these injuries, rare, minor, and fast-healing, are much preferred to the chronic injuries many of you suffer, or will suffer if you continue depending on shoes to protect you from bad running technique. So just watch where you step, and let your feet grow strong and healthy and free!

It is important to realize that conditioning of the feet is not simply a matter of toughening the soles to withstand the abrasive surfaces we will be running on.

Over the years, your feet have been protected from exercise by wearing shoes. Obviously, our soles will be over-sensitive at first. Therefore, it is very important to take plenty of time to strengthen, not just our soles, but also the entire foot structure. Focusing on learning HOW to run, instead of trying to build distance, at the beginning will also give our feet time to adjust, to strengthen, to regain a more natural level of sensitivity.

But physical strength, toughness, and conditioning, are way less important than retraining our mind. We will never improve our running technique, unless our mind is relaxed and open to listening to our newly bared soles.

Another important consideration is what types of surfaces we will be running on.

Each surface has different benefits. Soft, smooth, unlittered lawns, for example, are simply more comfortable to run on barefoot. However, soft, smooth, unlittered lawns, or rubber tracks, do little to condition the soles of our feet. But, they will help, to some extent, to strengthen the structure of our foot.

Hard and rough surfaces, while not all that comfortable to run on barefoot, are quite tolerable IF we use good running technique, and keep our joints fluid, not tense. These surfaces are great for developing and helping to maintain a wonderfully fluid, and relaxed running technique, which will help us on every surface we run on. So, while it isn't necessary to run exclusively on hard, rough surfaces, it isn't productive to avoid these surfaces either.

In the real world, you are going to run (hopefully barefoot) on all sorts of surfaces, dirt, grass, asphalt, concrete, granite mountain stream beds, hard packed clay, mud, rocks. While not all will be the most enjoyable, sometimes it's the variety that we can take pleasure in. Each type of surface, helps us with different facets of our running, technique, toughening the soles, or just learning to relax while running. Each surface provides a different type of massage for our feet. Don't be afraid to seek out and run or walk barefoot on each of the different grades of surfaces.

August 21st, 2007

Ken Saxton

What's your niche?

Why do we run on two feet? How is it that a big brained, hairless, weak, slow biped came to dominate its environment thousands of years ago? In this first chapter we will wrestle with some of these questions and in the process gain a better understanding of why, despite fashionable trends towards high intensity cardio, we truly are born to run long and slow.

Man is often called by laymen a "generalist" how else could such a puny animal contend with the massive ice age animals with which it competed for food? After all, man is a slow runner. The world record 100 meter dash speed is 10.02 seconds. That's roughly 37 Kilometers per hour sustained at maximum of 200 meters. In comparison, the fastest land animal, the cheetah can sustain three times that speed (over 100 K/h) for 1000 meters. There was little chance for us to outrun or outfight predators.

. Man is also relatively inefficient compared to its competitors. In a paper by David R. Carrier. Titled <u>In The Energetic Paradox of Running and Hominid Evolution</u> we find that while most mammals of our weight range expend roughly .10ml of oxygen per gram of body mass per kilometer of transport. We humans expend double that, nearly .22ml per kilometer.

So we are slow, relatively inefficient and physically weak. You might be asking, what possible niche a human could fit into in an environment full of massive, powerful and fast animals?

When our pre human ancestors first walked out of the forests on two feet in search of food, they probably encountered something similar to the modern African bush. At night, the African savannah would have been a terrifying place, with all manner of large pack animals preying on unsuspecting herds of ungulates with poor night vision.

During the day the bush was a much calmer place. The big cats, placated from a night of feasting would play lazily in the shade. Also hiding from the blistering heat of midday would have been our prey.

With shade in short supply, animals like Kudu would probably gather in predictable locations.

Even if a small, intelligent ape was able to track one of these walking feasts how does he go about killing it? For the early human hunter the midday sun would have been his most powerful asset.

As a cheetah, or any other animal runs, its core temperature rises significantly. Once an animal reaches a certain maximal core temperature it must stop running or risk heatstroke and sudden death. While a cheetah can run close to 100 K/h it can only do so for about one kilometer before overheating and stopping its chase. This is true too of our ancestor's prey.

Fur is an insulator. A furless animal, with its bare skin exposed to the wind would dissipate heat at a much faster rate than an animal whose primary form of heat dissipation is panting. Panting is inefficient, because it interrupts breathing and is only slightly more effective than heavy breathing.

So a large herbivore, while powerful, is much more subject to heat exhaustion than a hairless sweating Hominid. Scientific research also points to our special neurological abilities.

The literature argues that human sweat glands may be subject to a higher level of neuronal control than other animals. Principally due to the neurotransmitters used to activate the sweating process and the greater innervation of human sweat glands.

Understanding how important a hairless body is to our niche, one can immediately see the physical resemblance of our skin with other long range, hairless midday walkers such as elephants

This may all be old news to dog owners who like to jog with their pets. While a dog could easily out dash you, usually after some long, slow stuff, your dog is panting heavily and struggling to keep up.

Bipedal running, despite costing two times as much oxygen as quadruped running, has some distinct advantages when it comes to running down prey. All four legged animals have a tight 1:1 coupling between breaths and stride rate. Because of the physiology of four legged animals, They can only breath one time per stride.

This limitation means there is a specific combination of stride length and stride frequency that minimizes energy consumption. While a quadruped might be more efficient at a certain speed, it's drastically less efficient if pursued at a speed far less than that or at variable speeds. This is where bipedal predation becomes an excellent adaptation.

Standing upright on two feet instead of four, our breathing is unhitched from our stride rate. Allowing us to run at any speed and be equally efficient. A prehistoric persistence hunter could have run at its prey's most inefficient pace, while suffering no additional fatigue himself.

Average human running speed is roughly 8-10 kilometers per hour. For an animal to generate a breeze great enough for its fur to wick, it must run well over that speed. Being pursued by a human runner would not allow for animal to stop its dramatic rise in body temperature.

Hunting large efficient quadrupeds in the heat of the day requires seemingly supernatural heat dissipation abilities unrivaled in the animal kingdom. Its no surprise that no mammal is known to sweat as much per unit of surface area as man.

Our marathoners, able to run 26.2 miles in midday heat accomplish a feat that would kill any lion or tiger. Couple that with a brain so perceptive that it can anticipate and track animal's movements for days, and you've got a winning species.

Understanding our ecological niche allows us to train smarter. There is a current trend in the fitness industry to short, punishing, circuits and speed work. These HIT aficionados boast that, "boring" cardio is a thing of the past. They argue that primitive man was some muscular behemoth whose most respectable attributes would have been his brute strength and quickness, what a joke.

While no one doubts the strength of primitive man compared to his softer descendants, as Homo Sapiens range expanded beyond the savannah his superior intelligence and ability to work in groups is probably what made him master, not raw strength.

One need only compare human physical abilities to his environmental competitors to understand where we fit into the picture. Our ancestors relied on going long, not fast for food. If proponents of HIT think they're on the next big thing consider this excerpt from George Beinhorn

> *During the 1950s and 1960s, the top runners trained heavily emphasized intervals. But the interval-trained champions were soundly trounced when Arthur Lydiards runners came on the scene. Peter Snell, Ron Clarke, and Murray Halberg did just 6-8 weeks of speedwork, after laying in a 12-week base of pure aerobic endurance running. Runners who've done tremendous volumes. of speed work like Emil Zatopek and Bill Mad Dog Scobey couldn t match the times of the endurance-trained Lydiard athletes.*
>
> *-George Beinhorn*

HIT principles have been around a lot longer than the age of internet marketing, but they've still never caught on with the professionals. The training methods of elite runners are no accident. They coincide with our evolutionary biology, you'd better train like its 100,000 B.C. and that means building a strong endurance base over a period of years.

With that said, augmenting a dedicated endurance program with speed work can at the very least keep you from getting bored. In later chapters I will recommend some cross training activities to be done in conjunction with your regular program.

We just got well acquainted with the conditions under which your body evolved. Why is this important? Because it helps us train smarter. Having the belief that genetically, all healthy adults are designed to run over great distances is liberating.

You should expect great feats of endurance from yourself. Your ancestors, whether you're from Siberia or Nigeria, accomplished some incredible feats of mental and physical endurance so that you could sit here and read this. You're born to run.

This first chapter should also evoke some questions about why, if we are born to run, are there are so many injuries in the running community.

Now let's get into the meat and potatoes of this paper. In the following chapter we will talk about how modern footwear is inhibiting the amazing running machine that you are.

What is the purpose of running shoes?

The modern running shoe and footwear in general have successfully diminished sensory feedback without diminishing the injury impact, a dangerous situation.

~Robbins, Hanna

If we really needed all of that padding, why weren't we born with big puffy feet instead of the thin sinewy appendages that we inherited?

If you're reading this paper, then you've probably been asking yourself the same questions. Despite a surprisingly large scientific literature, very few people would see someone running down the street without shoes as a normal, healthy activity.

Western cultural norms that look down on being barefoot are fine when your out at a dinner party or working on a construction site, but when it comes to exercise, leave your intellectual laziness and at the door.

Your workouts should reflect the science, not the current fashions in footwear. Doing that means questioning the type of footwear that we use while training our bodies to become stronger and more efficient.

Let's begin with one of the most basic assumptions about current footwear: cushioning Shoe companies have poured a lot of money into research on their shoes ability to prevent impact forces from reaching the body.

Cushioning, Form and Tension.

It was found that, when running at moderate speeds, more than seventy five percent of all long distance runners make first contact with the ground on the heel part of the foot. However, the heel pad deformation of a barefoot runner would, after a few strides, fail conclusively to protect the heel from the high impact peak of a new running bout.

Each foot strike transfers approximately 2-3 times your bodyweight. To reduce these impact forces, shoe companies have attempted to bolster the padding of the heel. This would in effect accomplish what nature could not by increasing the cushiony stuff underneath your heel.

Shoe designers have effectively reduced the impact and accompanying discomfort caused by running in heel strike form. By increasing shoe padding, the heel pad can then deform more, reducing sensation and initial impact force.

Why wouldn't we want this to occur? Isn't it good to be comfortable? Actually yes it is.

If the human body is uncomfortable when heel striking barefoot, the solution is not to artificially alter the structure of the foot, but to allow the body to adjust itself naturally to a more comfortable running pattern.

Many of the laboratory studies that have lead to the current design of recreational running shoes focus on the first few seconds or minutes of a subjects running pattern. These critical first seconds reveal a large spike in the impact forces on the body.

This spike is particularly exaggerated in the barefoot condition. This initial spike is a result of the barefoot runners initial learning period, in which the runner would adjust his/her form to land as gently as possible. This correction of form in the first few steps usually results in something closer to a forefoot strike than the traditional heel strike.

In comparison, shod runners impact peak is less, but this lower initial force actually has detrimental effects. When any runner begins a new running bout, be they shod or barefoot, there is a great deal of involuntary activity occurring to protect the connective tissue from coming under too much stress.

Consider this excerpt from the Journal of Orthopedics and Biomechanics, which addresses this very phenomenon.

"When measurements are preformed on a limited number of steps, runners are able to sustain and then maintain high impact peaks, whereas in the present study the repetition of impacts induced by three minutes of running probably led the runner to reduce the high mechanical stress occurring at heel level. These mechanical adjustments are probably obtained by switching from rear to forefoot technique. Forefoot running is characterized by lower impact peaks and higher pre-activation of plantar flexor muscles."

The highly engaged or "Pre-activated" muscles help reduce injury and increase stride rate. EEG measurements are significantly higher in the lower foot muscles of a barefoot runner. The increased tension of the muscles allows impact forces to be dissipated without undue stress on the body.

When running in shoes however, the initial reduced impact peak and reduced sensation trick the brain into thinking its running on a uniformly soft surface. The tension reflex is greatly inhibited.

The shoe is unable to supply the adequate cushioning to compensate. As a result, the foot is less capable of protecting tendons and ligaments and there is an overall increase in the wear and tear on the body

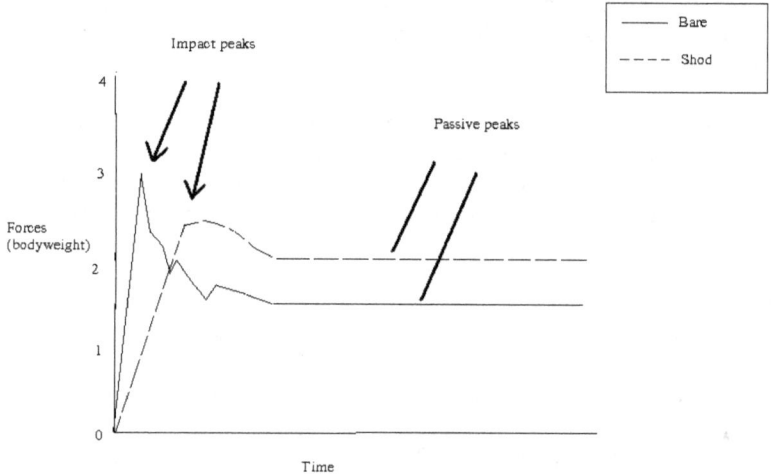

The higher passive peak found in the shod condition (the peak of force reached after steady running has begun) results in a greater incidence of injury over the course of a recreational runners lifetime.

Its also important to note that a barefoot runner will naturally alter the tension applied depending on how hard the surface she/he is running on to maintain a consistently low incidence of impact. Much like switching the gears of a bike.

However in the shod condition, the foot to ground connection is severed. The brain is tricked into thinking that it is running on a consistently soft surface, despite varying degrees of hardness. The result is that a runner will carry their poor form over a variety of surfaces, increasing incidence of chronic injury.

Footwear makes you less efficient

Your body's ability to efficiently utilize oxygen is an important aspect of running faster.
A less efficient runner requires more oxygen to move their body than a more efficient runner. This oxygen cost is a good indicator of who will be running the faster races, and reaching their genetic potential.

The weight of modern running shoes is the main detractor from running efficiently. It was found that an extra mass of just 100 grams per foot yielded a one percent increase in metabolic cost.

The addition of .5 or 1kg on the feet during sub maximal running leads to a significant increase in oxygen consumption. Considering the average pair of running shoes weighs about 677 grams/pair can you really afford not to run barefoot? That's a decrease of more than 6.5 percent in running efficiency. You need only look at your last race time and subtract 6.5 percent from it to see how dramatic this shift to barefoot running can be.

The nature of barefoot running form may also lend itself to greater overall efficiency Barefoot runners limit local pressure on the foot and increase leg stiffness. Running barefoot also results in a higher stride frequency, lower contact and flight time, lower passive force peak and a higher activation of foot muscles.

Although barefoot running is more physically involved, it is actually more efficient than running than the anesthetic environment of shoes.

Another reason barefoot running may be more efficient is due to the enhanced storage and restitution of elastic energy. This is probably due to the above mentioned mechanical adaptations. Also compared to shod running, barefoot running represents the natural means of locomotion. As a result the tendons and ligaments of the foot are properly used to store and release energy.

Going barefoot to reduce back pain

Many runners suffer from some kind of chronic low back pain. It may not come as a surprise that running induced low back pain may indeed be caused by overly cushioned shoes.

Like we said earlier, when the highly sensitive bare foot makes contact with the ground the body engages many impact mediating responses. To protect the lumbar spine from excess loading, the lower back engages an erector spinae muscle response.

Every time your foot hits the ground your body receives an impact equal to several times your bodyweight. With your foot contacting the ground for no more than a fraction of a second, hundreds of pounds of pressure can be exerted upon your body.

This quick transfer of force requires a quick onset of neurological tension to safely dissipate it. A quick reaction is the key to protecting the heavily loaded structure of your lumbar spine.

However, the dampening effect of modern running shoes greatly reduces the onset speed of the erector spinae and gluteus muscle responses.

This latency of response between the vulnerable structure of the lower back and the feet may be responsible for your chronic low back pain/discomfort.

The above mentioned effect can be best explained through a simple analogy. Imagine the force from the ground traveling through your body is like water flowing through a garden hose.

Every time your foot hits the ground, it's like you've opened the valve and water is flowing through the hose. At the other end of that hose is someone ready to squeeze the hose shut before the water escapes. If that person were given a delay of a second or two before they registered that the hose was on, some water will escape before they can stop it.

Stupid analogy, I know. But imagine that happening hundreds of times a minute, in the case of the hose you'd fill a swimming pool in no time. When it comes to your body that accrual of force might just create a chronic injury.

If you have nagging back pain, you may want to consider wearing thinner soled shoes on a daily basis. Kick off those shoes whenever you can and go barefoot, your back and posture may just thank you.

Should your kids be going barefoot?

I firmly believe this is the most important chapter in this booklet. Parents will agree, what could be a more important subject than the healthy physical development of their child?

A study comparing foot motion of children in shoes with unshod walking revealed that commercial shoes do indeed have a significant influence on the motion patterns of children's feet.

Like a grown individual, the natural gait of a child without shoes allows for complete flexion of all the bones and muscles of the foot.

However, unlike an adult there are greater implications to inhibiting the range of motion of a child's rapidly growing foot.

In a study by the University of Heidleberg, it was found that inadequate footwear or even footwear in general may affect the physiological development of the foot. In 2300 children between the age of 4 and 13 years the incidence of a flat foot among those who used footwear was significantly higher compared to those who did not.

Children wearing closed shoes showed a higher incidence for flat feet than those wearing sandals. Remarkably, only 36% of children had normal feet.

So, next time you're out buying shoes for your kids, consider this quote directly from the above mentioned scientific paper:

> *"The shoe should in no other way influence the normal foot than to protect it against lesion and coldness."*
> *-Foot motion in children shoes: a comparison of barefoot walking.*
> *Wolf S; Simon J; Patikas D; Schuster W; ArmburstP Doderlein L Gait*
> *& Posture*

Look at your own feet, is your pinky toe smashed up against your other toes like your wearing ballerina shoes? Or are your feet wide and muscular like someone who has never worn shoes before?

If we can convince even one parent to let their young child abandon their shoes and run around the yard barefoot, then this book was a success. Consider carefully the foot binding you are inducing next time you're tightly lacing up your toddlers shoes and the physical pleasure of running barefoot they may never experience.

Reasons The Kenyans Dominate Long Distance Running

Kenyan distance preeminence has nothing to do with genetics, but is a product of their environment and lifestyle. Before becoming a missionary in Uganda, L. Lantz graduated from Rensselaer Polytechnic Institute in 1992 with an E. E. degree and worked for Lockheed-Martin for 10 years as a systems programmer. This article contains his findings from three years of observation in East Africa and from his own running experience there.

I have lived in Soroti, Uganda for the last three years with my wife and six children. I am 37 years old and am a Baptist missionary. My town is approximately 125 miles from the Kenyan highlands. I currently run 40+ miles barefoot here in East Africa each week. It took me about six months to toughen my feet up to where I can do this. I have done several 12 milers barefoot and have experienced no foot/ankle problems. My daily runs take place on a dirt road. I began on grass but became tired of stepping on corncobs (they throw those things everywhere). I am not super fast (19:05 5K at age 34). I am not some barefoot running weirdo, but I simply want to increase my weekly mileage and I was getting countless knee and ankle problems from my shoes.

Living here has taught me many things about the runners that East Africa produces. There are many reasons why they perform better, and not one of them, I believe, is due to genetics.

Why The Kenyans Dominate
1. School. East African children walk and at times do even paced running to/from school each day. Not one child is ever driven to school. Less than 1% of the population has cars. A child must come from a rich family to have a bicycle before age 15. Kenyan children begin laying down a solid aerobic base beginning at age seven. (Note: Many don't graduate high school until age 21).

Here is a weekly schedule:
• Mon-Fri (in elementary years): 2-3 miles in AM + 2-3 miles for PM run.
• Mon-Fri (in Jr./Sr. high years): 3-6 miles in AM + 3-6 miles for PM run. (There are fewer Jr. high + Sr. high schools. They have to run farther to reach them.)
• Saturdays: soccer workout.

• Sundays: rest, maybe a little soccer.
Many children add a third cardiovascular workout each day by digging in the gardens for an hour before they go to school. When school is out for holidays: children enjoy more soccer and running and walking to visit neighbors in nearby homestead or villages. These kids will have an 8-year aerobic base developed by the time that most U.S. teenagers complete their first year of track and field!

2. Soccer. There is only one sport for most of Africa soccer. Soccer gives each runner his weekly speed workout. Soccer allows these children to keep in touch with their fast-twitch muscle fibers as they build their aerobic base. The directional changes during soccer games and practices really strengthen the leg tendons and ligaments needed for hard running workouts in the future.

3. Barefoot training. 99.5% of East African children run barefoot for the first 14 years of their life. Benefits:
  a. Barefoot running allows them to develop proper running technique.
  b. No knee and ankle injuries due to bad shoes. They don't have problems with uneven shoe wear, as their shoes never wear out. There are virtually no overtraining issues.
  c. No training injuries due to obstacles. When a barefoot runner steps on a rock or in a hole, the torque is much less for a barefoot person than for a person wearing a shoe with a one-inch heel. (Note: I have stepped on a few racquetball-sized rocks while running barefoot and have been able to run the next day. If I was wearing shoes, I would have definitely turned my ankle and needed to sit out for a day or two.) Perhaps the best thing barefoot running does is keep injuries to a minimum.

4. Lower foot strength. Barefoot running strengthens foot and lower leg muscles to an incredible degree. You simply would not believe how much stronger your ankles and feet become. All other things being equal, I believe 15 years of barefoot running give the average Kenyan an extra 5% edge with better running economy and closing speed. I am continually amazed at how much explosive power I see in these young children as I see them sprint around barefoot. Looking back in my life, I think only 10% of the kids I grew up with in South Dakota had that kind of speed/power by that age.

5. Recovery is faster. Barefoot running does not stress the major muscle groups as much. Since I have begun barefoot running, I have noticed how my quads have shrunk. Barefoot running does not engage the big muscle groups like shod running does. I can do a hard two-hour barefoot run and not have tired quads or hamstrings. When your quality runs become longer than one hour, your hamstrings tire simply from pulling your shoes through during each stride.

The quads also tire as they try to balance out workload by adding a little more forward propulsion. Since the weight of a running shoe is all at the extreme end of the lower leg, it requires a good deal of force to propel it along. (This is because of the added torque---e. g. try to lift a sledgehammer to a horizontal position by gripping the handle on the extreme end. It's very hard, because all of the weight is at the extreme end of the moment arm.) In barefoot running, however, the big muscle groups do not become as tired. The calves and feet do the brunt of the work. The entire stress of the workout is placed on the cardio system. Thus, recovery is faster for the Kenyans.

6. Higher intensity workouts. Barefoot running allows more trapped heat to be thrown off during a workout. Energy normally expended trying to dissipate heat can instead go to the creation of new capillaries in the legs and the strengthening of the heart. Most of the time the ground is much cooler than you would think (through morning dew, or nighttime rains). Grass is cool even when the sun is out. When running on grass, the feet are continually cooled throughout the workout. I can constantly achieve much higher heart rates during workouts with less discomfort when running barefoot. In my experience, my level of effort to achieve an 84% MHR barefoot seems to equal my effort to achieve a 78% MHR shod.

7. Cooler workouts. The workouts of Kenyan runners take place in the mountains. The morning temp in East African Mountains is probably 60 degrees year round. We are on the equator so there are no seasons of winter, spring, summer and fall. (Every day of the year, the sun comes up at 7:00AM and goes down at 7:00PM.) They have perfect training temperature. Because of cooler temperatures, the body has to do minimal work to throw off the accumulated heat during a workout. I believe the more energy that can be put into running (and the less energy and blood that is recruited to cool off the skin) the better the workout will be. I would think an athlete would want the heart working hard to create new capillaries in the legs, instead of being taxed to push the blood to the surface of the skin to cool the body off. Also Kenyan workouts do not have to be adjusted due to ice or snow in winter or due to hot, humid weather in July and August. Thus Kenyan mountain weather is unmatched as far as training climates go.

8. Athlete selection. Kenya's fastest and most gifted young athletes do not drift into sports (like baseball, football, tennis, gymnastics) that stifle the ongoing development of their aerobic base. All of Kenya's best young athletes engage in one sport-soccer. And they run, run, run.

9. No extracurricular activities. There are no jobs for teenagers, and no other sports or after school programs to conflict with their training. You would never have an athlete say "I only have an hour to get in my afternoon run." American teenagers spend a great deal of time in extracurricular activities. Kenyans do not. I know this will sound lame, but in East Africa, even girlfriends are not in competition for the athletes' time. In East African culture, a man does not date girls until he is at least 21. In my tribe the age is closer to 22/23 years. This is because the duration of courtship for marriage (in most cases) is less then one month, and even then the young man needs to hold down a suitable job if he is to marry a young woman. You may think this is an irrelevant point, but the environment in Kenya makes it much easier for athletes to engage in 7-10 year training programs. The result is athletes who end up competing on the international level, not guys who just want to make it to the state finals in high school. There are simply not a lot of things competing for their time.

10. No high school track programs. Kenyan teenagers do not have the two or even three track seasons each year like U.S. high school runners. (They may have an occasional race or two, however, against another school.) Thus they have nothing which would interfere with their base building phase. Their base building phases are not shortened as with U.S. track and field athletes.

11. Their diet. In short, they don't drink soda or eat junk food. Because of the high cost of soda, the only time they drink it is at Christmas and at weddings (trust me on this). They eat no ice cream, sugary cereal, pop-tarts, twinkies, ho-ho's, cool-aid, popsicles or candy bars. Their diet consists of rice, beans, bananas, millet, and carrots. The only time they eat meat is at Christmas, Easter and at weddings. Their diet keeps them very lean. I think 90% of all adult men in my tribe have a waist size under 32 inches. Being so lean keeps them from running injuries. When you are 130 lbs instead of 150 lbs, the impact on your body from long distance running will be less. Thus you can train harder and are less likely to succumb to training injuries.

12. They have more patience. This is a cultural thing. In Africa, time has little value. (Again, trust me on this.) For instance, one hour late for an appointment is OK and no apology is normally needed. The East African runner is way more patient than his American counterpart. Kenyan teens don't need or demand the immediate results that U.S. kids want. They don't stop running because they are not hitting their goals. They don't switch to hard track workouts to catch up for missed years of laying down a proper aerobic base. They are not looking for a quick fix. They don't burn out.

13. Absence of interval-minded coaches. Kenyan children train in the absence of track coaches. They don't have a crazy coach who thinks his athlete needs to run more and more intervals. As a result, they do not suffer the ill-fated injuries of so many high school runners in the U.S. Instead, the Kenyan runner continues to build an impressive aerobic base of 7-10 years and remains injury free.

Conditioning the soles of the feet

How to best condition the soles of the feet continues to be a controversial issue.

Long time bare footers claim that little break in is necessary if ones form is perfect. Others struggle for months, even years with blisters aches and pains.

On the subject of protecting your soles, the best consult is Barefoot Ken 'Bob" Saxton
Who has run an astounding seventy marathons barefoot!!. He says:

> **"Some surfaces are more conducive to blister formations, but that depends on how the foot is interacting with the surface. If you are getting blisters on ANY surface, then either your foot is skidding, twisting, spinning, or otherwise sliding on the surface - or you are running too far, too fast, too soon (which is also a function of HOW your feet are interacting with the surfaces - ie: you are not ready to run very far, because you still need to learn HOW to run gently).**
>
> **Make sure your foot is landing on the surface, at exactly the speed the surface is moving under your body. Likewise, simply LIFT the foot off the surface, as it travels backward behind your body. Do NOT try to push off, or do anything else that causes the foot to slip on the surface.**
>
> **No matter how smooth the surface, do NOT do anything that would cause undue pain or injury on a rough, hard, pointy surface.**
>
> **No matter how rough the surface, think as if you were running on a surface covered with wet paint, and didn't want to slip, slide, or twist in the paint. No matter how soft the surface, distribute your weight across the entire sole of your foot.**
>
> **Ken Saxton**

The greatest protection from blisters comes in the form of prevention. Practicing good form on dry ground will reduce most of your blister problems.

Good running form is inextricably tied up with properly protecting your feet. Modern surfaces are much more uniform than anything you might encounter in nature. This is both a blessing and a curse. While roads and racetracks offer a clear surface and little chance to roll an ankle they can also have a shearing effect on the soles of your feet.

This sandpaper effect will quickly wear into any skin that is dragging along the ground. As a beginner is important that you learn to land and lift your feet with a minimum of shearing.

Try to focus on bending your knees down toward the ground as you lift your feet rather than pushing off with the balls of your foot like a sprinter.

The padding underneath your big toe is most prone to blistering because beginning runners have a tendency to push off as they finish their strike. Instead, land on the outside of your foot and roll your feet gently inwards so the padding underneath your big toe is the last to receive the grounds impact.

When it comes to good running form it is absolutely imperative to relax all of the muscles in your body. Your body knows reflexively the right amount of muscular tension to apply to a given surface, it's your job to relax into proper form.

While exact foot placement is a personal choice, landing gently and quickly lifting your foot WITHOUT pushing off is imperative. Let your weight fall forward instead of trying to push off with each stride.

Most barefoot runners run with a mid-foot stance, because the mid-foot strike allows you to dissipate the most weight evenly without having to use the heel to push off or the toes to pull forward.

To help elicit good running form, try to lead with your hips rather than your feet. By leaning your torso forward you let gravity propel you forward. Running then becomes a matter of catching your body with bent knees, while quickly "kissing" the ground with your feet.

With that said, your stride rate will be much greater when running barefoot. Often all that's needed to decrease the blistering and cracking of the soles is to increase your stride rate while maintaining that same gentle form.

You might want to consider counting your foot turnover per minute. If you run with a watch all you need to do is count the number of times a single foot touches the ground in one minute then multiply by two.

A lower stride rate usually indicates that you're propelling yourself foreword by pushing your feet off the ground. Or that you're dragging your feet before your lifting them, which increases contact time with the surface.

You should shoot for around 175 gentle contacts with the ground per minute or more. For some that might seem like an awful lot.

Initially you might feel tired, and in the beginning it will be difficult to concentrate on moving your feet at that speed for a thirty or forty minute run.

While the less uniform surfaces of trails or paths may allow you a slightly lower foot turnover. To ensure you are properly protecting the soles of your feet, it's important to train yourself early on to maintain a quick stride rate.

Remember that every training run is a neurological experience. Your body remembers every workout good and bad. So be sure you take the time to learn good form from the get go. Check your stride rate often when you're beginning.

Remember:

1. Tip forward, lead with your hips

2. Land mid foot, on the outside of your foot

3. Gently roll toward the big toe before lifting your foot

4. Lean deeper and increase your stride rate.

Lower Leg soreness

Lower leg soreness is almost universally felt when a runner switches from shod to unshod running. Particularly if that runner is disposed to forefoot rather than midfoot or heel striking technique

Shoe companies would agree that the function of the shoe during running is to provide a soft, but stable structure which in theory allows for a protective dampening to occur between ground and foot. This cushioning is exactly why most shod runners never feel that wonderful "lighting up" of the lower leg muscles, especially the muscles surrounding the Achilles, namely the soleus muscles.

By connecting his/her foot to the ground, the barefoot runner is creating a neurological chain from the sole of the foot to the brain. The runner is allowing the body to make the necessary corrections in running form to account for terrain changes. More subtly, the body is also making alterations in muscle tension.

Muscle tension and leg stiffness caused by muscle activation in anticipation of footfall is one of the primary means of protecting the joints and skeletal structure.

The level of neurological activation of the Gastrocemius and Soleus muscles are noticeably different between barefoot and shod runners.

Most heel to toe runners delight in "resting" by leaning back on their steps, stretching out the Gastrocemius muscles and letting their heels fall like a hammer. The result is over stretched underused muscles.

Stretched out soleus muscles receive such a jolt of neurological activity from the snapping movement in unshod running, that a beginning runner can become quickly fatigued.

Even those shod runners who run with minimal cushioning are failing to properly activate the lower leg muscles.

The barefoot runner naturally changes muscle tension according to the surface encountered. By covering the foot at all, you effectively trick the brain into the wrong muscle tension to ground impact ratio.

 In effect, the only way to train the lower leg muscles to respond properly to the ground is to "teach" the muscles of the lower leg to activate at their optimum by going barefoot more and more on many different surfaces.

Incorporating barefoot running into a program

If you're a fairly dedicated runner, it's probably likely that your current endurance outweighs the durability of your bare soles. This means that you probably will not be doing all of your running barefoot at first.

There are many ways a runner can incorporate a barefoot running into his program. In this section I will mention just a few tried and true methods on how to keep you running while adding mileage barefoot.

The three run per week beginner program

In this program your training is centered on three runs per week. With a day break in between each run for cross training and rest. (Monday, Wednesday, Friday would be run days, Tuesday, Thursday, and weekend would be cross training and recovery)

Each run in this program is specifically designed to train a particular aspect of your endurance. It's extremely important that you write down the results of each run to ensure you are reaping the benefits.

Run #1: The long run

On this day, wherever you choose to place it in your training week, you will run the longest. The purpose of this day is to log miles and train your aerobic system. Go slower than your normal pace by a few seconds at least every mile.

The exact number of seconds you should trail by is relative to your current goals and mileage I wont go into the exact science on how you should pace your long runs. That information can be easily attained elsewhere. However as a general rule you shouldn't be going all out on your runs.

Run #2 Your tempo run

The purpose of this run day is to set your pace for races, it's typically 3-5 miles for 10k and 5K races, For longer races this run is usually between 8-10 miles.

On this day you should be setting the pace for the race ahead, however in the case of the barefoot runner, do not compromise form.

Run #3 Your speed work day

On this day you should be focusing on speed during a given event. It is not recommended to run this day barefoot as the track repeats you will be doing could tear up the soles of your foot, particularly in the case of the beginner.

Shoot for a pace somewhere around your fastest five k pace. Most speed sessions total about 5000 meters done in increments of 400-2000 meters interspersed with rest.

To train for speed you're going to want to be consistently fast throughout your speed work session. Try to maintain a constant speed rather than burning out in the beginning of your session.

A three day per week program that stresses aerobic capacity, tempo, and speed work allows a runner plenty of room for training barefoot and performing a desired cross training activity.

It should be pretty clear where one might fit their barefoot training into the following program.

Perform light barefoot running during cross training and rest days until you can run 3-5 miles confidently, then begin running your tempo runs, or part of your long runs barefoot.

Your times may drop slightly during the transition from shod to barefoot. Just focus on maintaining perfect form while running barefoot.

Mixing Miles: for the more advanced

Those who have already laid a significant mileage base or wish to break away from the more rigid format of the three days per week program may want to consider Mixing Miles.

Mixing Miles is a simple concept that lends itself perfectly to incorporating barefoot training while still maintaining a big mileage base.

The beauty of Mixing Miles is that you customize the number of miles you run each day, ensuring that you maintain a weekly minimum.

Say that you run 35 miles per week, rather than run five miles every day,
you could run
15 on Sunday,
1 mile on Monday,
10 on Tuesday,
3 on Wednesday,
Rest on Thursday,
6 on Friday,
And rest again on Saturday

For a total of 35 miles per week.

For the dedicated runner who wants to keep things interesting, this type of training has definite benefits.

It also lends itself very well to incorporating a barefoot running regimen. Take a look at the number of miles run on Monday, just one. Perfect for loosing the shoes and doing some light barefoot work.

Again on Wednesday, just three miles. A relatively short distance to run barefoot even for a beginner.

In a few months one could also run Fridays six miles barefoot.

An experienced runner could throw in more light barefoot work or cross training on Saturday or Thursday.

Mixing miles allows you to craft an intuitive program. You will begin to get a sense of how long your feet need to recover between barefoot runs.

You can change you miles accordingly, slowly taking miles from your long run and distributing them amongst your barefoot sessions until you have worked up to an impressive barefoot mileage!!

Cross training

Cross training is an important aspect of any runners program. It promotes recovery while working the same muscles as running. It also prevents boredom.

Some of these activities require more skill than others. You should try to practice your cross training workout at least two times a week on off days of running or on days when your mileage is very light.

Here are a few common cross training activities that might compliment your training well. These workouts fit in well with the three day per week beginner program, but may be replaced as your mileage continues to increase.

Swimming

Swimming is an excellent non-impact way to improve overall fitness. Not only does it increase upper-body strength and endurance, but it takes stress off of the legs. Swimming increases the flexibility and strength of lower leg muscles as well, important for a barefoot runner.

Swimming requires much more technique than other physical activities. Work on moving comfortably and efficiently in the water before you try to build an endurance base.

Here are a few tips for barefoot and shod runners who are interested in increasing their running performances. From the Furman Institute of Running and Scientific Training.

- Rather than swim with a fast arm turnover strive to keep the strokes long and relaxed. Distance per stroke is more important than number of strokes per minute. Concentrate on getting as much distance per stroke as you can. Try to reduce the number of strokes you take per lap

- Try to develop good breathing technique remember to exhale completely with your face still in the water before rolling your head to the side to breath. If you find that you are getting out of breath quickly, ask a swim instructor to offer some tips on your swim stroke.

- Since runners are accustomed to using their legs for propulsion many runners who start swimming kick to hard. Swimming is primarily and upper body activity, since kicking provides around ten percent of the forward propulsion.

Bicycling

Bicycling is a non weight bearing low impact aerobic exercise that develops aerobic fitness while allowing you to recover from running.

Furthermore, performing speed work with a bike can help increase leg turnover, which is a definite plus for barefoot and shod runners alike.

Although cycling is an excellent way to perform cross training, it can be expensive to purchase a good bike, and is often dangerous in foul weather and on busy roads.

Sport

Regularly engaging in soccer, basketball or any other team sport is an excellent way to boost your speed, and increase your endurance base. Moreover the playful aspect of sport means it's a welcome refresher from a long slow day of running.

The main focus on this book is transitioning to a barefoot running program. Be sure not to let these activities hamper your main goal of transitioning to a complete barefoot running program.

Weightlifting

To specify the exact forms or amounts of muscular exercise advisable would take us beyond the scope of the present work. Here as elsewhere the student must work out his own salvation
-The Ministry of Muscular Activity to the Body as a Whole Published 1906

There is such a vast knowledge on the subject of weightlifting it would be impossible to include all of it within this paper. Luckily, when it comes to lifting weights you needn't know everything. Ill focus on some tried and true methods to becoming a stronger, faster runner.

If you think weight training will make you bulky, think again. Becoming a bodybuilder is no accident. The huge metabolically inefficient muscles that bodybuilders carry around require enormous quantities of carbs, fat and protein. Many bodybuilders consume 10,000 calories a day to maintain their shape. That needn't be you. If you want to be a strong, sculpted and fast runner you should be training with weights.

This book emphasizes natural movement patterns. Lifting a barbell is better than using a machine, and lifting dumbbells is the best because it allows your body to move in three dimensions rather than on a fixed plane.

Your body wasn't designed to perform perfectly symmetrical machine like movements over and over. The more fixed the object the more likely you are to develop a repetitive stress injury. By training with free weights we allow our naturally unsymmetrical bodies to make minor adjustments and bring usually neglected muscles into play.,

While free weights may seem harder at first, rest assured, the payoffs in strength will be tangible. Notice how much less weight the average gym rat can bench press when he is using dumbbells as compared to the conventional Olympic bar.

If you're training for athleticism, you need to work your body in a coordinated manner. How can you expect to perform better athletically if you never train your nervous system to work in unison? Stick to a few compound movements that force the body to work in concert.

Dead lifts, presses and other full body exercise train intramuscular coordination very similar to that of the sports you play or the things you do in everyday life. That's why it is said these exercise develop functional strength. Doing functional movements will allow you to run faster, jump higher and move with more coordination. this is particularly important for barefoot runners whose bodies are more heavily engaged in running than their shod counterparts.

You should work your entire body in each session. When you exercise your entire body, you release the maximum amount of growth, repair and maintenance hormones. It's also more efficient. Working your entire body in each session requires that you train only every other day.

So how much should you lift and for how many reps?

As we said before the primary goal of your training will be an increase in strength. When training for strength, it is helpful to think in terms of your one repetition maximum or 1RM. Your 1 RM is the amount of weight you can lift just once on a given exercise, such as the Deadlift.

Calculating your one rep max:
- Set #1 Do 3 to 5 reps with a weight which will not allow you to perform a 6th repetition. Rest for 2 minutes.
- Set #2 Do 2 to 3 reps with a weight that will not allow you to perform a 4th repetition. Rest for 3 minutes.

Set #4 Add 20% more weight to the bar and try to perform a single rep. You can manage more than 1 repetition rest for another 3 minutes, load the bar with slightly more weight and try again. Remember, you goal is to perform 1 rep only.

All repetitions should be performed in a slow and controlled manner, no jerking the bar off the ground.

Once you've determined your 1 rep max you should aim to lift 80% of that for two sets of five repetitions. (2x5) this might not seem like much muscle pumping, that's because it isn't. Keeping weight high and reps/sets low allows us to build tremendous strength without overtraining the muscle or adding bulk. Lifting heavy for few reps can actually reduce your chance of injury. Most injuries occur when you are mentally and physically fatigued and begin to let your form slip. Training heavy for few reps keeps you focused on hammering out quality reps in good form and then walking away before you get sloppy.

Training with near maximum weights forces your body to recruit more fibers during effort, this increased neuromuscular connection coupled with sport specific activity (such as running) will allow you to apply more force to the ground with each step, carrying you further.

Relative strength is an important aspect of increasing your overall athleticism. 175 pound athletes who can dead lift 3x bodyweight will always outrun the 300 pound athlete who can only dead lift 1.5 times bodyweight. Increasing your ability to recruit fibers is similar to upgrading your engine while keeping the same chassis.

With that in mind you should pick lifts that use the most muscle fibers in concert. Think dead lifts, squats, bench presses, overhead presses, and pull-ups. You needn't fill out your program with bicep curls and shrugs. For pure strength one only needs a few big compound movements

Olympic athletes have been known to train exclusively with the dead lift and a heavy press as their only slow grinding lifts. Obviously you want to minimize time in the weight room and maximize time running. That's the best way to improve. So hit the gym for some heavy Deads then head off for a run!!

Exactly what weight routine you choose will be up to you, just make sure your working your entire body each session and increasing either reps or weight lifted.

As always make sure your executing each movement in PERFECT form. Every time you hit the gym your training your nervous system to remember the movement patterns you perform. Be sure to ingrain proper form early on, or suffer the consequences.

For a complete exercise database with accompanying form videos visit http://www.exrx.net/index.html

It's an excellent resource to increase your knowledge of healthy training practices.

On to the structure of your weight training.

A tried and true method for increasing strength without hitting plateaus is called periodization. periodization refers to breaking up your exercise program into a series of periods, in each period you work up slowly to a new personal best over a period of several weeks before de loading to a new, higher starting point. Here's an example of a typical period progression

Workout Number	1st Set Weight		Reps	2nd Set Weight		Reps
1	200	x	5	180	x	5
2	205	x	5	185	x	5
3	210	x	5	190	x	5
4	215	x	5	195	x	5
5	205	x	5	185	x	5
6	210	x	5	190	x	5
7	215	x	5	195	x	5
8	220	x	5	200	x	5
9	210	x	5	190	x	5
10	215	x	5	195	x	5
11	220	x	5	200	x	5
	225	x	5	205	x	5

As you can see, this athlete approached a new PR in the dead lift by cautiously approaching, then backing away before overtraining occurred. A sort of two steps forward, one step back approach.

Try to plan training cycles to last between 8-12 workouts, after you've hit a new record or you feel like you're physically too trained to push for a new PR, simply begin a new progression.

This simple and effective weight training program will innervate your muscles, and get you breaking plateaus of strength for years to come. But remember, as a beginner you will see drastically more improvement than you will a year out.

There is a point of diminishing returns in any activity that requires you to apply skill over a period of time. While an advanced weightlifter may only add 5 pounds in a year, a beginner may add 70 pounds or more to their dead lift using this same method.

There you have it folks, an effective way to recruit and build muscle that eliminates the pointless muscle pumping most bodybuilding routines call for. Follow this program, and you'll be a stronger runner in no time.

Almost Barefoot

What about those of us who want to shed our old running shoes altogether? There are alternatives for people who don't have sunny warm weather 365 days of the year. These barefoot alternatives will keep you on the road in foul weather while still maintaining some of the benefits of barefoot running.

Vibram Five fingers

The Five Fingers is a form fitting Vibram soled running shoe that has captured the hearts and minds of many bare footers. Not surprisingly, this shoe has also caught on with those who were not mentally ready to run barefoot, but still want to walk the walk hoping to get the best of both worlds.

This shoe has benefits for runners who wish to continue strengthening the muscles used in barefoot running during the foul weather seasons. However the thick Vibram sole has the unfortunate effect of dampening the sensation of the ground. As we learned earlier, the body cannot compensate properly for impact forces without the foot actually touching the ground.

Your form will be sacrificed by wearing these shoes. Moreover after a few weeks you may find yourself developing aches and pains where there were none previously. Compared to running barefoot, you will have much less spring in your step. as a result you will hit the ground less gently.

To test just how much less recruited your muscles are compared to the barefoot condition, you need only affix a five finger shoe to one foot and go barefoot on the other.

The difference is dramatic, and the shoes drawbacks are apparent.

However, as a walking shoe, the Five Fingers is just about the most comfortable around. I would recommend this product as a daily use shoe to anyone beginning down the path to barefoot running. You will find it succeeds in strengthening and stretching the feet where other shoes fail.

Furthermore this shoe confers all of the postural benefits of barefooting, by allowing the foot to rest flat on the ground without raising the heel.

The Five Fingers flat bottoms also make this shoe ideal for weightlifting. While lifting heavy objects off the floor without shoes is by far the safest, the five fingers allow you to grip the ground in much the same way. You may find yourself lifting more in these shoes.

Aqua sox

Aqua sox have become another popular form of minimalist running footwear. These super cheap foot coverings allow you to feel even small pebbles. Most don't last remarkably long considering the material their made of, but they will usually suffice for a winter or two of running. You can find variations of these beach shoes and other waterproof socks for as low as five dollars online.

This section is intentionally brief. When you find yourself searching for barefoot alternatives remember that there is no magic pill when it comes to running barefoot. To truly reap the rewards of going barefoot and to call yourself a true barefoot runner, you must run barefoot.

The above alternatives are still excellent choices for those who wish to reap partial benefits of reduced footwear while protecting the feet from harsh weather.

Putting it all together: structuring the perfect program

Today's mighty oak is just yesterday's nut that held its ground.
- David Icke

Designing a specific training program without knowing your specific goals would provide little value to you. In this section we will look at two hypothetical training progressions,

Runner #1
Joe is a beginning runner who wants to train to run a 5k Barefoot,

Runner #2
Sally is a more experienced runner looking to retain her mileage while reaping some of the benefits of barefoot running.

===========================
Runner #1

Joe decides to pick the beginner three day per week program to reach his goal of running a 5k barefoot.

Because he's a beginner, Joe has a very small aerobic base. He picks a 5k race 12 weeks away to allow for adequate buildup.

Next, Joe plans out his first few weeks based on the three run per week method. Because Joe has never run a 5k before he isn't quite sure what his race pace will be. To determine his race pace, Joe goes to his local track and does an all out 5k.

Now that he has an idea of the time and distance he will be shooting for, Joe sets up his tempo run to match those goals.

Because Joe's relatively untrained, his speed work will be light to begin with. Every week he runs a few 400 meter intervals with rest in between. Slowly adding intervals every week.

Finally for his long run, he runs more than his target race distance (5K) but much slower.

Joes first week of training looks like this.

Monday
Speed work: 2 x 400 meters with a cool down

Tuesday
Light barefoot training, ran one mile.

Wednesday
Tempo Run: 1K warm-up 3K at target speed 1K cool down

Thursday
Barefoot run on trails, cycled to work

Friday
Long Run 7K at 7 minutes slower than race pace.

There's plenty of room for Joe to incorporate barefoot running wherever he can. While gradually increasing the distances run in each of the three main running days.

=========================
Runner #2

Sally is no beginner. She has been running consistently for six months and now averages about thirty five miles per week. However whenever she tries to push her mileage higher, her feet begin to ache and she backs off her training.

Sally decides to break her training up like this:

Monday
3 miles barefoot

Tuesday
10 miles

Wednesday

Rest, lift weights/swim

Thursday
10 miles

Friday
7 miles

Saturday
1 mile barefoot

Sunday
Rest. Lift weights/swim

After a few months mixing her miles, Sally has gradually increased her mileage on barefoot days and during her long runs. Not surprisingly that nagging pain in her feet is a thing of the past.

A challenge to our readers

Let me just say congratulations on taking the first step towards running barefoot and thank you for supporting this fledgling project!

If you bought this book your now part of a tribe, it is the authors intention to grow this book to meet the demands of that tribe.

Ours is a small tribe. As a first edition reader your comments and questions are extremely influential on how this tribe will grow and develop.

You are now more knowledgeable about barefoot running and human biomechanics than 99% of the population. It is your job to point people in the right direction. Use this book as your guide.

If you have any questions on biomechanics or on any of the information within this book please email us.

As interest in barefoot running grows, I look forward to your continued involvement in the community. I encourage you to find other barefoot runners near you to organize running clinics and run races together.

Just think about what a positive impact you'd have in the world if you convince even one parent that their child should go barefoot. And as a result that child's foot develops properly.

I want you to envision yourself running races barefoot, surrounded by those whose minds have yet to be opened.

Envision yourself bringing into question the notions of those shod runners around you as you confidently pass them.

Knowledge is contagious

If you can inspire even one person to read this book, then you've helped grow this community.

You've eaten the red pill, let's see how far down the rabbit hole goes.

Conclusion

The intended purpose of Barefoot Running, Complete Course is not to provide a quick gimmicky solution to your well intentioned desire to run naturally. Nor is the intention of this paper to teach you to run according certain method or rigid form.

This paper should be read as an accumulation of knowledge on the topic of barefoot running. Consider this book a lecture in print on barefoot running and human biomechanics rather than a perfect no fail system that promises to reduce all your injuries instantly.

The object of this paper is to instill a running for life mentality coupled with a strong knowledge of how to begin a solid running and bare footing program.

Ultimately proper calibration of your program must come from you. Only you can know exactly when you've run too much or too little.

I encourage you to use the information contained within this book as a knowledge base from which you can craft your own intuitive program.

I think you'll be pleasantly surprised, even after years of shod running how quickly your body provides for you proper running form and response.

By reading this book you've made the first and most difficult step toward running barefoot. Have fun and good luck!!!!!

The doors of Barefoot-Tribe.com are open to you. We are always open to those who are walking the path and have legitimate questions or comments on how we may improve this paper and the knowledge within it for future editions. Or how we may improve the community as a whole. (Or if you just have a barefoot running success story you'd like to share)

Please contact us at
Brn2runsuggestion@gmail.com

Works Cited

This book is just the beginning.

Below is a list of the primary sources used in writing this book, I encourage you to continue your study into human movement and barefoot running. I don't pretend to have all the answers. It would be impossible to fit into a single paper all of the wisdom accumulated on the subject of barefoot running and human biomechanics. Use these articles to get deeper into the subject. Never rest on your laurels. Expert status awaits those who continue to learn and relearn. Good luck and have fun!!!!

1. Journal of applied biomechanics, Stiffness adaptations in shod running. Divert C; Baur H;

2. International journal of sports medicine, Mechanical comparison of barefoot and shod running. Divert C; Mornieux G; Baur H; Mayer F; Belli A

3. Journal of biomechanics, Biomechanical analysis of the stance phase during barefoot and shod running. De Wit B; De Clercq D; Aerts P

4. International journal of sports medicine. Barefoot-shod running differences: shoe or mass effect? Divert C; Mornieux G; Freychat P; Baly L; Mayer F; Belli A

5. International journal of sports medicine. Footwear affects the behavior of low back muscles when jogging. Ogon M Aleksiev AR; Spratt KF; Pope MH; Saltzman CL

6. Gait & Posture. Foot Motion in Children shoes: a comparison of barefoot walking Wolf S; Simon J; Patikas D; Schuster W; Armbrust P Doderlein L